FROM FAT TO FIT

The Weight Loss Steps to Success

Table of Contents

INTRODUCTION

My book has found its way to you, and I want to start by thanking you for acquiring it. I invite you to join me on a journey that is going to transform your body. You must now choose to follow the path that has been placed before you if you genuinely wish to improve yourself and lose weight. Along the way, there will be several obstacles you will need to overcome. I will provide you with all the tools you need to overcome them. You will have triumphs and failures. Your success will not be defined by your perfection in following the steps in this book. Your success will come by your willingness to get back up when you fail so you can learn from your mistakes and avoid repeating them. Only then will you find what you seek at the end of your weight loss journey. I believe this book can help almost anyone shed a significant amount of weight. I am living proof that it works.

My Story

I'm not a bodybuilder, an athlete or a health professional. I don't get paid to be fit, and I am not in perfect shape. So, you might ask yourself why you should take my advice. Like a lot of us, I work behind a desk sitting down all day. Like most people, I split my time between work, family, and entertainment. I was overweight for the last 20 years of my life, so I know firsthand how hard it can be to lose weight and the challenges that await you. I also believe I represent most of the population who don't have the time or the inclination to go to the gym for hours every week. By following the 7 simple steps laid out in this book, I managed to lose over 100 lbs. So, if *From Fat to Fit* worked for me with my history of obesity, I believe it can work for almost anyone.

When I started my journey, I was 260lbs. It was in 2012 when I was at the peak of my obesity. I didn't care about the food I ate; I did not care about my body, and I hated my reflection. I was fat and depressed, plus I had back pains and severe digestive issues. I had no energy, and I had no love for myself or for my body. Folks would see my double chin, and I could see the disapproving looks in their eyes, and it made me ashamed of myself. All these problems were all related to one thing: I was out of shape, big time. One day, I woke up and my back hurt so much I could barely get up. Lying in bed that morning, an image of a morbidly obese person came to my mind. This man was on a TV reality show, and he was so heavy he could no longer walk. They had to cut the wall in his home and get a crane to bring him to the hospital. I saw myself heading in that direction. That morning, I decided to start a new path, and without knowing it, I started the first step on the road to my weight loss journey.

From that day forth, I started doing things I had never done before.

I discovered new foods to eat and experimented with new techniques. I tested several different approaches to figure out the best way to lose weight. This book is a compilation of the seven major factors that helped me lose 100 lbs. and become fit. I created these steps after examining my own weight loss journey. They represent my own series of actions that brought me to my new healthy body.

Today, I am proud to say I am fit and pain-free. My back and digestive problems are gone, and my energy level is higher than it has ever been. People now look at me with respect in their eyes; they see me in a different light. I love how others see me now and how I see myself because I am proud of my reflection. I am healthier and happier than I have ever been. You can be too if you choose to follow the steps.

From Fat to Fit

You need to follow the instructions below to work with the steps

- The book is divided into seven steps.
- You must complete each step one at a time.
- Once you have fulfilled the challenges, you can move on to the next step.
- You must continue to apply the previous step as you move on.

You won't have to count calories or points. It is a straightforward method, allowing you to spend more time losing weight and less time doing the math. Some diets might state you can lose a massive amount of weight in a short amount of time. In some cases, this might be possible, but what's the point of losing 30 lbs. in a month if you gain it all back next month? The truth is, losing weight will take some time, but by taking the long road, you give your brain a chance to adapt, and that gives you the advantage of increasing your chances of keeping your weight down.

Take your time and work on each section until you have completed all the challenges; it is that simple. Throughout this book, I will cover some necessary information, some of which you might already know. I believe it is essential to include the basics facts because we tend to overlook them, yet they can have a massive impact.

Accepting Change

Your success may depend on your willingness to follow every step along the way. Each chapter has some essential information that must be integrated gradually so your mind can become accustomed to each one. It's necessary you complete the challenges at the end of each step. This will ensure you have completed everything and grasped the concepts. You may think you will achieve quicker results by going faster, but losing weight takes time and must be a gradual process. If you rush, you will be overwhelmed because the brain does not accept change readily. Here are three things you should never do to avoid overdoing it.

- Do not skip any steps.
- Do not go to the next step until you have done all the challenges.
- Do not attempt to do all the steps at once.

The mind has one area that handles new tasks. A separate section of the brain is for habitual actions. Your mind is wired to think and act as you have in the past. When you try something new, your brain will decide to reject it, like an intruder. It will come up with all kinds of excuses.

- I worked all day; I should reward myself with some TV time instead of exercising.
- I walked on Monday, so I do not need to do it again today.
- It is raining outside today; I'll go biking tomorrow.
- I haven't lost any weight; this is not working.

You must not let these thoughts convince you to stop, but don't ignore them either. Instead, you must recognize these as the brain's self-defense mechanisms to any new change. The mind tends to defend itself against the unknown since this is a fundamental fear we all share. Once you understand this, it becomes easier to put these thoughts aside and push forward with each new step. Use your intelligence to recognize you are not under attack. Bypass this self-defense mechanism by identifying this new change should be perceived as a friend coming in to help, not an intruder.

Some steps might be hard to handle at first. However, as you work on them every week, you will find they will start to become part of your routine, and your mind will begin to accept them. At this point, your task will move to the habitual part of your brain, making it easier for your conscious self to complete them. Almost anything can move from one side to the other. Just give it some time and be persistent.

Weight Loss Benefits

Losing weight has many benefits. Being fit is not only about looking good and being healthy. It's also about being proud of your body and feeling comfortable within yourself. It's important to love yourself when you see your reflection. To have the capacity to walk up a flight of stairs and not be winded. To feel young again and have a body that can follow you on new adventures and experiences. No one wants to have pains and aches every day, causing you to feel trapped in your skin, never able to do the things you dream of and only seeing them experienced through others on television. No one should suffer this fate. Fitness will free your body and enable you to experience anything your heart and mind desires.

Losing weight will transform your body into a healthy, well-oiled machine. You might live longer as a direct result of this. As you might know, several diseases are directly related to obesity, thus shortening life expectancy and quality of life. By completing all 7 steps, you will lose weight, giving yourself a better chance to avoid many painful, deadly diseases such as heart disease and strokes, high blood pressure, diabetes, cataracts, gout, osteoarthritis, gallbladder disease, nonalcoholic fatty liver disease, pulmonary diseases, phlebitis, severe pancreatitis, idiopathic intracranial hypertension and several types of cancers.

If you are in a relationship, your spouse might be more attracted to you as you lose weight. If you are currently single, it might become easier to find an attractive partner. It is important to remember we attract who we are. If you are positive and in shape, you will attract such people to you naturally. Think about these benefits when you are going through challenging times.

The Motivation Goals

Before you start your first step, I want you to think of the main reasons you want to lose weight. Your motivation goals are something you want to do, accomplish or have once you are in shape. Take a few minutes to write down all the goals that come to mind. Even if they seem ludicrous or impossible, just do it. Below are some examples of goals.

1. Climb a mountain.
2. Go to the beach and not feel ashamed to take off your t-shirt.
3. Wake up without any backaches.
4. Fit in that old pair of jeans.
5. Meet a new partner.
6. Combat an on-going disease.

Writing them down will help you visualize them so you can make them happen. This way, you will create a vision of your weight loss. Feel free to add pictures or drawings. During tough times, read your motivation goals to get you back on track. I decided to take a big 2 x 3 ft cardboard and write down all my motivation goals. It's on my wall in my office, so I see it all time. When I get demotivated, I take a minute and read through it all. It helps me regain focus and motivation. Read your goals as often as possible; they will keep you centered and focused on the path to weight loss. They are an excellent source of motivation to remind you of all the things in life you want to take advantage of.

You are about to embark on the first step of your weight loss journey. Open your mind to new experiences and possibilities. Raise your standards of what you expect from yourself. Your thoughts, body, habits, and behavior can all change for better or for worse. It is up to you to choose which one. Don't let any negative thoughts infiltrate the fortress of your hopes and dreams. Anything is possible if you keep at it every day and believe in yourself.

STEP ONE: SUGAR

As a child, I loved sugar. Ice cream and candy were often my rewards for being well behaved. I have fond memories of making a few dollars for doing some chores and then running to the convenience store and buying my precious candy. I would spend all my money to fill my pockets with my favorite kind. In my teens, I drank my share of soft drinks daily. As I grew up, I accepted this tasty treat as something good and natural, something that made me happy. But I was deceived.

I now know sugar can be more addictive than cocaine. It's the primary cause of obesity and diabetes. Holidays like Halloween, Easter and Valentine's Day have been twisted to perpetuate the selling of more chocolate and sugar. It's become a corrupt substance added to almost every food it can get into. We are addicted to this substance virtually from birth. I see videos of toddlers stuffing their faces with birthday cake, and it makes me sad to realize most children are given processed sugar with no afterthought of the consequences. The bottom line is it's a toxic grain, a form of poison that makes you fat and sick. It must be avoided at all cost to succeed in your weight loss journey

The sugar cycle must stop. You must take your first step towards a healthy body and say NO to white sugar. When you understand white sugar is a slow poison, you will find it easier to start letting go of it. Therefore, the first task is to eliminate it from your daily consumption. Removing sugar is no easy feat, but it's essential to your weight loss success. I will guide you through the process.

White Sugar Elimination

It's important to note that when excessive amounts of sugar are consumed, your body converts it directly into fat. Your body then stores fat as a system to keep you fed and alive in case food becomes scarce. In today's world, we rarely run out of food, but our body does not care; it's programmed to store extra calories for later. When later never comes, it just keeps accumulating more and more fat. Therefore, it's essential that you stop consuming white sugar today and control your sugar intake to avoid gaining extra fat. You must stop adding more fat on before you can start to lose the fat you already have. I have put together a series of tasks to help you accomplish this:

1. Start by eliminating your single most significant source of sugar in your life right now. For me, it was soft drinks. I used to consume enormous amounts of cola. I could easily drink four to five cans a day, if not more. That is about 200 grams of sugar a day, which is about five times the amount my body could process. So, I started eliminating soft drinks from my daily consumption as I understood this was my most significant sugar intake. I stopped buying it and

11

poured out what was left of my cola in the sink. I found the hardest part was when people offered me some at parties. I merely smiled and declined and asked for a glass of water. It was hard at first, but I ultimately felt much better after a few weeks, and I never looked back. Examine your weekly eating habits and your grocery list. Find out which sugary food comes up the most for you. Once you know what it is, stop consuming it entirely. If you have some in your fridge or pantry, get rid of it and throw it in the garbage or pour it down the drain. Eliminating your biggest sucrose foe is crucial to your success. Recognize that food is meant to nourish your body, not to poison it with fat and diabetes. See this as a challenge; you must overcome this obstacle in your quest to attain a healthy body. Give it time, and its hold on you will disappear. Remember, you decide what you put in your mouth. Don't let food control you. If need be, give yourself a few weeks to adjust to this new task before moving on.

2. Once you have eliminated your most prominent source of sugar, the rest should be much easier to remove. You now need to stop consuming any food item that contains excessive amounts of added sugar (this includes candy, soft drinks, juice, cake, etc.). Most foods have a white label with nutritious facts on it. Make a habit of always looking

at it for every item you buy to find out how much sugar it has. Only buy products that have fewer than 5 grams of added sugar on the label; ideally, there shouldn't be any sugar. You need to be able to identify the other various sources of sugar around you. You can get it in a raw form such as brown sugar, white sugar or powdered sugar. It's in many products we know today: chocolate, cookies, ice cream, candies, juices, soft drinks, cakes and more. Sugar is also added to certain foods you might not expect like bread, pasta, and sauce, just to name a few. Read the labels on the processed foods that you buy to see if any white sugar has been added to it.

3. You should avoid places where the target is to sell you sugar. Pastry, donut and candy shops are good examples. At the supermarket, don't walk down the row where all cakes, baked goods, and soft drinks are. The more you stay away from them, the easier it is to stop eating them. Try to locate other food outlets and stores in your area that don't sell as many sugary products and visit them instead.

4. Abstain from keeping any sugary products at home or at the office. The more there is around, the more you want to eat it. Get rid of it and resist the temptation to keep any at all. Don't hide sugar in your home or make a secret stash of

sweets; this only serves to weaken your resolve. Remember your goal, and keep it in your mind, always.

Replacing White Sugar

Like any drugs, the more you take, the more you want. When you quit consuming white sugar, you might suffer some withdrawal symptoms. You might get headaches or experience some mood swings. It might be even worse if you are consuming substantial amounts of sugar every day. Therefore, you need to replace white sugar (sucrose) with fruit sugar (fructose). This will help fill the void and help fight off your addiction to the white grain.

There is a difference between sugar found in fruits versus soft drinks and fruits juices. Fruits contain sugar, but they also provide, minerals, vitamins, and fibers. The fiber in fruits has two parts to play. First, it slows down the absorption of sugar. This effect moderates the impact on your blood sugar levels. Second, because of the fiber, fruits are digested slowly, giving more time for your body to use that energy. However, when you drink something sweet or eat candy, your pancreas secretes insulin to deal with all that sugar at once. Over time, your cells can become resistant to insulin, and this leads to diabetes and weight gain.

When you get a craving for something sugary, replace your sweet treat with your favorite fruit. When you have the urge, you might think of a soft drink, chocolate or candy. It differs from person to person, but when you break it down, it's only a craving for sugar that you have. The need you have for cookies or ice cream is just the hidden addiction to sugar. When you eat fructose from fruits, it sends the same satisfaction message to your brain. The difference is that fruits won't make you gain weight. So, eat them until you are satisfied. Wait 15 to 30 minutes, and the sugar craving will vanish.

Eating Fruits

To begin eating fruits, find a place nearby your home and make it a weekly task to stock up on fresh fruits. You can buy them at any supermarket, but open markets and fruit stores tend to have better deals. Fruits vary in price based on the season and geographical location. If you go to a market, you can usually buy them in a more substantial quantity at a low cost.

Before you eat any, find out what is the best and easiest way to prepare them. It ensures you enjoy the fruit and will, in turn, motivate you to discover new ones. A quick search online will demystify this for you. I would go over them now, but thousands of different varieties of fruits exist around the world today, so I will let you determine this on your own. Fruit is nature's candy, and some may be a hidden pleasure waiting for you to discover.

There are several periods during the day when it is easy to incorporate fruits into your diet. Breakfast is one of best times to eat fruit, as it gives you a boost in energy and your body can use it to power through your day. It can also help to prevent afternoon sugar cravings. During the afternoon, eat an apple or a banana for a quick and easy snack on the go. Fruits can also make a beautiful dessert. Mix some melon, pineapple, and oranges and toss them in together for a delicious fruit salad. They can also be added to plain yogurt to replace white sugar. Always have fruits in the fridge and on the table, so when the time comes to eat, they will be highly visible, and you will have easy access to them.

Fruits I Recommend

There are thousands of types of fruits, each one has some health benefits. Try different ones and see which of them work best for you. All of them are good for losing weight. The important thing is choosing the ones you enjoy the most, so you will continue eating them. I have listed the sugar content of each fruit, so you may compare it with some of your white sugar products. Some say you should avoid overeating high sugar fruits, but I will tell you that a higher sugar content will help you overcome your sugar cravings more efficiently. If you don't know where to start, here is a list of the most common fruits you can find almost anywhere.

Citrus Orange: They are a reliable source of vitamin C. There are about nine grams of sugar in each orange. This will help you cope with the loss of white sugar. They also help combat the formation of free radicals that lead to cancer. They are loaded with fiber, which will help to keep you full longer.

Filling Bananas: They are delicious and cheap. Eating one keeps you full for an hour. They contain loads of potassium, which is essential for fighting off muscle cramps. They also require no washing or preparation of any kind. There is 14g of sugar in one banana.

Dessert Berries: All berries are great for desserts and shakes. They are sweet and tasty. The most known are probably strawberries, blueberries, and raspberries. They are excellent for breakfast along with some eggs or in a bowl of cereal or oatmeal. Strawberries and raspberries have 7g of sugar per cup and blueberries have 15g.

Lean Apples: They have a compound called polyphenols in them. It attracts good bacteria in your gut associated with weight loss. They have a high sugar content, so they are a great weapon to use against sugar cravings. Apples can be mixed into a salad or washed and eaten on the spot. It is better to eat them uncooked since heating them destroys the polyphenols. Apples have 19 grams of sugar per apple.

Sweet Grapes: They are lovely and have a high amount of sugar, which makes them a top choice when getting an intense sugar craving. They are also known for their anti-oxidant properties. As a bonus, they also help prevent cancer, diabetes and heart disease. You can quickly eat them as a snack or mix them up in a salad. Grapes have 15 grams of sugar per cup.

The fruits above are only suggestions. I recommend you try them as well as new ones of your choosing. Stop eating any you dislike and try others. Test and eat as many kinds of fruits as you can get your hands on and stick to the ones you like the most. Always keep a variety of about 3 to 5 different fruits in your kitchen. This variety ensures you do not get bored when it comes time to eat.

After a few months without refined sugar, you will notice some changes. Your body will start to transform. You might have more money in your pockets since you wisely spend it on some healthy choices instead of expensive sugary products. You might also find it easier to avoid white sugar. The cravings for candies and ice cream will be replaced by a desire for health fruits. You will have more energy from consuming fruits and less of a down from sweets.

The Challenges

1. Stop eating your most significant source of sugar.
2. Remove all remaining sources of white sugar.
3. Avoid places where their primary target is to sell you sugary products.
4. Abstain from keeping any sugary products at home or at the office.
5. Replace white sugar with your favorite fruits.

This step should take approximately a month to complete. It might be longer depending on the depth of your addiction. Don't rush into it; positive change takes time. If you barely eat any sugar, this will probably be a quick and easy step for you. Even if you fail at times, remember that success is not determined by the number of times you fail but the willingness to get back up when you do and to keep going. Make sure you have completed the challenges above to the best of your ability. I know this is not easy but believe me, it's worth it. Once you have completed the five challenges mentioned above and kept up with them for at least a month, you will be ready to move on to step 2.

STEP TWO: WALKING

Once you have neutralized your sugar demon, you will be free to begin losing weight. The second step in your journey from fat to fit is to go out and start walking; it's that simple. The goal of this step is to take five walks a week, and each of them should be a minimum of one hour.

Your walks can be done at separate times during the day. For example, you can walk 15 minutes to go to work in the morning, go for a short 30-minute walk during your lunch hour and finish it off with a 15-minute walk back home at night to complete your one hour. If you are overthinking and haven't gone walking today, just step outside right now and start walking in any direction. Even if it's just a few streets from your home, the critical thing is to get into the habit of walking every day.

Walking Goal

Have a goal in mind when you go for a walk. This will help you stay motivated, so you can complete your daily ritual. Your objective can be something as simple as going to the grocery store and coming back or walking to your friend's house and back. It's always best to estimate how much time this will take, as you want to aim for the one-hour mark. Use Google Maps to calculate how much time it will take to get from point A to point B and then back. This is also an efficient way to find parks, trails and other places you might want to go. Remember, your goal should be something simple.

Motivation

Get into the habit of bringing your cell phone or your camera to take a picture of yourself or of something unique during your walks. It could be some street art on a wall or a cute snail you decide to save on the road. Whatever it is you enjoy about your walks, take a quick picture. It's a smart way to remember the good times you had along the way. Some days, you might be tired, and you won't feel like walking, and that's normal. During these times, you can look at the pictures you took on your walks. They will provide you with a positive source of encouragement to go out and walk the earth.

Walking is one of the best exercises you can do to lose weight and keep it off. As a matter of fact, our entire body is made to walk. It's designed to do so every day, and it's by far the most straightforward exercise. Compared to other activities, walking is safe to do whatever your weight is. Even if you have a lot to lose, there is almost no chance you will get hurt. Therefore, walking comes as the first exercise you should do to start losing weight. It can be difficult or painful to do any other sort of prolonged activity when you are overweight, so stick to walking until further into this book. Otherwise, you could end up injuring yourself and postponing your weight loss. Plus, the beautiful thing about walking outside is that it's free. It's an excellent way to start working out as several other types of exercises require expensive equipment or memberships.

When the sun is out, take advantage and use it to motivate you to go out for a stroll. The sun is a great morale booster; it provides you with a good dose of vitamin D. This vitamin is good for fighting depression and can make you naturally happy. This feeling will become a positive addiction as you actively seek to walk in the sun. Use this to your advantage to stay motivated to go hiking in the light. Think about it on the days when it's harder to get up and move; think about how warm and happy you will feel when you will be walking in the sunlight.

Benefits of Walking

Walking makes your body stronger. It improves the bones and muscles in your legs and makes them stronger. Your legs have the most powerful muscles in your body, and thus they require the most calories to activate. Just like any muscle in the body, the more you use them, the stronger they get. Your body is automatically maintained by walking. It can prevent or manage serious health problems including heart disease, diabetes, and high blood pressure. Your body is a lot like a car; it needs to stay in motion, so everything can flow properly. If you don't walk enough, you will start to break down, and no one wants that.

Walking is also excellent for your mind. It allows you to be alone with your thoughts and contemplate the people in your life, your current job, and any events that are happening to you. When you walk, you will notice you think and reflect naturally. In a sense, it's a form of meditation, and it can help you discover great insights that will help you resolve problems. After you have been doing it for a few months, you will find it hard to go a day without your hour-long adventure.

Treasure Hunt

You can find all sorts of things while on your walks. One day, I was walking back from work on a long straight street in the suburbs. It was a grey, windy day; humidity hung in the air as if it was about to rain, but it never did. Tall green trees lined the street like Roman pillars. As I got to the end of the road, I looked to my right. Lying on the ground, I saw a twenty-dollar bill on the driveway, next to the sidewalk. Just like magic, the wind brought it there for me. What are the odds, I wondered? I was feeling depressed and lonely that day, and it's like the universe sent that money my way to cheer me up. I was genuinely amazed, and part of me wasn't entirely convinced it was real. I was sure it was a fake, so later, I asked a lady at a store to verify it for me. She confirmed it was real; I couldn't believe my luck.

A few months later, I was taking a walk downtown and found an expensive watch. It was lying on the ground waiting for me to pick it up. It was ideally placed on the side of the road like someone had left it there for me. I found later it was worth close to a thousand dollars. I still have it to this day, and it's a reminder of what walking has brought me.

During your walkabouts, you can find all kinds of free loot all over the place; look around you, and you might spot some. Among other things, I have discovered sunglasses in the woods, a wrench, a lot of loose change and many other things. You never know what you will see when stepping out your door. Don't be ashamed or feel bad to pick up anything you find because otherwise, someone else will. Go out with an open mind, and you will attract positive things to you naturally.

The Simple Beauty

It's time to go outside and explore the world around you. Take a deep breath and appreciate this time you have put aside for yourself. There are thousands of places around you today that await your discovery. When you are walking, take time to appreciate the beautiful sights around you. You may not even notice the beauty that surrounds you every day when you zoom by it in your car. Step outside, breathe in the fresh air, feel the sunlight on your skin and enjoy Mother Nature.

There are plenty of places to visit around you right now. For example, nature offers us the best locations to explore: serene forests, beautiful mountains and flowing rivers filled with life. Outdoor experiences can often be the most memorable ones: seeing a spider make its intricate web or a small squirrel peaking its head through a tree. They can bring you inner peace with the realization that life is ever present everywhere around you.

If you prefer to avoid local wildlife, cities are great for sightseeing while walking. This goes without saying as millions of people travel to different cities every year, but it's also important to explore your own little corner of the world. Find out if there are any unique events happening in town and walk through them. You will be surprised at all the things you can observe in plain view. You might see a beautiful statue you had never noticed before or some exciting street art on the side of a building. Exploring on foot gives you the time to look around more thoughtfully and appreciate your surroundings. All cities have a life of their own and are an excellent choice for your daily stroll.

Time of Day

You must discover your favorite time of day to go walking outside.

Each one has its own merits.

You should try walking in the morning, the afternoon and at night to find out what time of day works best for you.

Walking in the morning feels great. You're up early with the fresh air. Once it's done, you will have more energy for the rest of the day and your workout will be done. In the afternoon, the sunlight is at its strongest and illuminates everything. Rivers sparkle like they are made of diamonds and the birds come out to sing amongst the trees. It's beautiful. At night, the darkness changes the atmosphere completely. The city lights come out, and from a high vantage point, it looks like a sea of stars. In fact, I used to walk a lot at night; I would walk in the suburbs past midnight until sunrise sometimes. There was no one in sight, no sound, only me, the wind and the moon. It's like walking in a ghost town like I was the only person left on earth. During that time, I needed to be alone with my thoughts and reflect on my life.

Nowadays, I prefer to walk in the sun where there are people and life all around me. At various times in your life, you will find you are drawn to the darkness or to the light; they both have their parts to play. Once you have found your time, keep to it until you find yourself longing for something else.

Finding Time

Between work, family, and friends, it's hard to find the time to go for a stroll every day. There is a time for everything, so do your best to find a spot in your busy life for your daily walk. If you are having trouble finding the time, here are a few ideas to get you going.

1. Instead of driving to the store, see if it's close enough for you to walk to. Stores are closer than you imagine. Use Google Maps to confirm the distance on foot. To carry your food back home, don't rely on cheap plastic grocery bags. Nothing ruins a beautiful walk like a bag getting ripped halfway in your walk. Instead, bring a backpack and 2 solid heavy-duty bags to make sure they don't collapse on your way back home.

2. Walk to work if you can or park your car further from your job and walk for 30 minutes to get there. You will save money on gas and complete your walking objective for the day. Also, by parking further away, you might be able to find a free area to park.

3. If you have kids, bring them to the park and play, walk and run after them. This is a fantastic way to spend time with your children and get your one hour done.

4. Dogs are excellent companions and will also require you to go outside and get moving. Your dog will be so happy when you bring him out, and it will help you stay motivated. You will have the responsibility to take him for a walk every day, and in turn, you can get yours done as well.

5. Going strolling around town is an excellent idea for a date with your girlfriend or boyfriend. Find a quiet park or a charming street in the city where there are people and music.

6. If it's raining, go to the mall or a museum. Keep walking around and try not to stop too often. This is an excellent trick to keep up your walks, even if the weather is terrible.

7. During your lunch hour at work, have a quick bite to eat and then go for a walk. Going for a mid-day walk will let you relax and melt off some stress. You will loosen up, and at the end of your stroll, you will be ready to head back to work feeling refreshed.

8. If you take the bus, find what time it arrives, then walk a few stops instead of waiting for it to come. The same can be said for the train. If it comes in 10 minutes, take this

opportunity to walk along the platform instead of standing still or sitting down. Not only will you get some of your walking time completed, but you will also transform wasted time into productive activity.

9. Always take the stairs instead of taking the elevator. This might seem like a trivial exercise, but if you do it every day, it adds up in the end.

Preparing for a Long Walk

When you are getting ready to go out, you can bring some water or perhaps a healthy snack like an apple or banana. You will spend some energy while walking, so eating a healthy snack halfway into your walk will give you a boost of energy to make your way back home. Bring a bottle of water if you are going out for more than one hour. You lose a lot of power when you are dehydrated. This is optional, but I recommend it if you are not accustomed to walking for extended periods of time.

This might sound obvious, but before going out for a walk, you must always check the weather for the next hour. This is a factor you want to take into consideration when you are preparing to dress. Do you need to bring your sunglasses and put on your shorts or should you wear jeans and carry an umbrella? These are simple questions you want to answer before you step out the door.

Weather can change sporadically from day to day, or from one hour to the next, so make sure you check right before you leave.

You must always be prepared when you go out, rain or shine. You want to avoid a situation that will make your time outside uncomfortable. The storm is a challenge to overcome. If you are well prepared, walking in the rain can be enjoyable. It brings its own soundtrack of thunder and lightning. The rain trickles down on every surface, and like a symphony, it plays for you. A beautiful sunny day always seems so innocent, but it can bring its own hazards. Getting a painful sunburn that lasts for a few days might dissuade you from going out in the sun again. Always wear sunscreen under that bright blue sky to avoid a negative experience. Being prepared will save you a lot of grief and will motivate you to go back out in the future.

The Challenges

1. Walk 1 hour per day, 5 days a week.
2. Take a picture during each walk.
3. Find the best time of day to go on your stroll.
4. Always be prepared before you go out.

Walking every day will take some time to get used to. Remember, the mind does not accept change quickly. You must let this settle in gently because it's a substantial change to your daily routine and it is essential for your weight loss journey. It will keep you moving and active. Once you have done it consistently for 1 month, you are ready to move on to step 3.

STEP 3: THE CALENDAR

This third step is about keeping a record of your progression and learning from it. The calendar is the written record of your development. You will create a training calendar and write down your physical activity you do every day. Whenever you go for a walk, or when you do any form of exercise, you must write it on your calendar. You can then use that information to find your weak points and to improve them. You will also discover your strengths. This can be a source of motivation. Think of your calendar as a map that can show you the way through a dense forest. It can reveal the path you must take, but only you can choose to follow it.

Working with the Calendar

First, print one out for this month. You can use a standard yearly calendar, but make sure it's only used to track your progress. Ideally, try and keep it somewhere private so only you can see it. This is merely to avoid other people's input on your progression.

Second, identify the calendar with the title like walking, training or exercising. Add some color to the borders to better distinguish it; I chose brown. You can even draw on the side or add stickers. How you decorate is up to you, but make sure it represents something positive for you.

Third and most important, get a red, green and blue marker and a black pen. Keep these nearby the calendar. Every day you go for your one-hour walk, make a green square around the date. In it, use the black pen to write down what you accomplished that day. For example, you could write: *I walked downtown for one hour.* If you did something extra, like 2 walks in one day, make a second square with the blue pen. This will serve as a visual reminder of the extra work you were able to complete that day. When you don't do any exercise for one day, make a red square around the date. As before, use the black pen to write down the reason you didn't exercise.

It's easy to forget when you have exercised, so the calendar is there to ensure none of your efforts are overlooked. Remember to fill it out every day to avoid forgetting what you did. Don't worry if you forget for a day or two; it happens to everyone. Fill out the missing information as soon as possible to have the most accurate calendar. Ideally, write what you have accomplished as quickly as you finish it. This will give you the highest feeling of satisfaction.

Honesty is essential for the calendar to work correctly. It's forbidden to write lies on it, and even if you do, you're only deceiving yourself. Don't be afraid to put a red square; it will help you to grow and improve. Once you do, more green squares are sure to come soon. Failure is a part of success, something that most people have trouble accepting. No one is perfect, and every single person will have ups and downs. The critical thing to remember is to always learn from your past mistakes so you can improve your future. If you can do that, your failures will only be part of your greater success.

Green Squares

Once a week, read what's written inside the green squares to appreciate the effort you've put into them. Also, look for patterns in the green and see if anything emerges. For example, you might see that you managed to walk home from work every Friday. See if you can make it a weekly habit.

The goal of the green squares is to track your progress and make sure you complete your 5 walks every week. Once you have earned some green squares, see how many you can get in a row. Challenge yourself to improve each month. Like a positive addiction, you will seek out the satisfaction it brings. Each green square represents a step forward in your journey to attain your weight loss goal. It embodies your on-going success in this fight for fitness.

Red Squares

You will get some red squares, but they are nothing to worry about. It takes courage to put them on the calendar. It must be done for you to learn your behavior pattern towards exercise. Laziness is not always the culprit behind lack of physical activity. You can't exercise every single day, and it's not under your control. Unforeseen events or demotivation can happen in life, and they can cause you to miss a day. The goal of the red squares is not to punish you. They will show you why and when you didn't exercise. With his information, you can discern if it's a onetime event or if a pattern emerges. For example, red squares often come up on the same days of the week. That doesn't mean you have to eliminate any weekly activities or events that prevent you from working out. Most of the time, there are solutions to work around them.

At the end of each month, I want you to review your calendar and read all the red squares you find. Focus on the reoccurring reasons why you missed exercising. See if a pattern emerges, so you can identify what triggers them and find an appropriate solution. Here are some examples of red squares and solutions:

1. *I missed my walk. I finished work and went to the bar.*

   Solution: Friday came up a few times during the month as a red square. One solution could be to get up early in the morning and go for a walk before you leave for work. Therefore, at night you are free to go drinking with your buddies. Another solution would be to walk back home from the bar.

2. *I didn't go walking today because it was raining.*

    Solution: The weather can be crazy sometimes, and you might not always feel like going outside for a stroll in the rain. Go walk into a shopping mall and clear your shopping list or go to a museum and walk around for an hour.

3. *I was too tired after work to go for a walk.*

    Solution: You might look at your calendar and see that on Mondays, for example, you tend to fall asleep on the couch when you come back from work. Next Sunday, go to sleep earlier so you are not so tired Monday evening and can go for your walk.

4. *I went to my friend's party.*

    Solution: Plan when you know an event is coming up. It's your friend's party so prepare to exercise earlier that day. Avoiding putting it off to later at night when you might be too tired.

5. *I had to go to the hospital for a medical emergency.*

    Solution: Some red squares are unavoidable, like a medical emergency. Very rarely will your calendar be completely green. You must accept that some squares will be red, and that's ok.

Remember, use the calendar as you would a map. It can guide you on the path to building better habits. It's a fantastic tool to motivate you to work out and walk more. It shows you a colorful visual record of your progression. You can look back on it and see all you have accomplished. As you progress in the system, you will have additional challenges that will fill out your calendar with green.

The Challenge

1. Print out a calendar and decorate it to suit your own taste.
2. At the end of the day, make a square around the date in the appropriate color and write what you have done or why you didn't.
3. Always be honest when writing on your calendar.
4. Once a week, read your green squares to help you stay motivated.
5. At the end of each month, look at your red squares and try to find solutions to them.

Your calendar is your badge of honor, your trophy, your gold medal, your everlasting proof of success. By reading *From Fat to Fit*, you have chosen to take a big step towards self-improvement. Remind yourself of that when you look at your calendar. You should be satisfied that you created it, no matter how much green or red it has. Be proud of your green squares and learn from the red ones. If you can keep it green, you will keep your body in shape. Once you have completed your first month, you can move on to step four.

STEP 4: THE FAST

On this fourth step, you will be doing a water fast for 32 hours. Based on my personal experience and research, I have found that fasting is the most efficient way to lose weight. It's the most significant discovery I made on my quest to attain a healthy weight. It tipped the scale in my favor, and it has become the greatest weapon in my on-going fight against fat. It's an essential step towards achieving your weight loss goal.

You might think fasting is something you would never do. The truth is, you're already fasting for about 8 hours every day. You dream during this time, so it's easy to overlook, but sleeping is fasting. Hence, when you wake up to eat your first meal, you have breakfast. The name itself states the nature of the meal: to "break" your nightly "fast." On this fourth step, I will merely ask that you extend that regenerative cycle for another 24 hours.

The Fasting Process

I will teach you how to complete a water fast. You must refrain from eating for 32 hours. During this time, you can only drink water, hence the name. The goal is to intake zero calories. When you break it down, it's only 16 hours because you are asleep for the first and the last eight hours. During the 16 hours, it's vital to keep drinking water.

Essentially, you are replacing solid foods with water, so you need to drink throughout the day. It will help avoid headaches, dizziness, and most importantly hunger. H_2O is the only liquid you can consume during the time, but you can drink as much as you want, so always have a full bottle with you. Make sure to bring your water bottle with you wherever you go, such as when you are out for a walk or shopping. Drinking will make you feel temporarily satiated because your stomach will fill, creating the illusion you have eaten, thus helping you fight off hunger. At some point, you might understandably be fed up with drinking water, but you should never stop. It could cause a return of your appetite. Instead, try to drink slowly, taking small sips more often.

It can be hard to stay motivated and to keep going without food. The key to completing your fast is to keep yourself distracted. Entertain yourself by doing things you enjoy. Play video games, watch television or read. Fasting is also an exciting time to let out your creative side. Try painting, writing or drawing; you might be surprised by the inspiration you can get when you are fasting. I know some of you are busier than others or have different obligations with children, work and everything else. Try your best to carve out this time for yourself at least once a month. Choosing an appropriate day to fast is vital for its success.

For your first fast, I recommend you take one of your days off and plan a quiet day at home. The countdown to 32 hours starts when you go to sleep the night before. For example, let's say you plan to fast on a Saturday. You go to bed at 11 Friday night and wake up at 7 Saturday morning. At this point, you already have 8 hours done. As soon as you get up, drink a tall glass of water to start off your day. Remember, you cannot eat until 7 am Sunday morning. Come Saturday night, near the end of the fast; it might be hard to resist the temptation to eat. At this point, remind yourself how much you have sacrificed today and how little time there is left to succeed. You might also be tired and out of energy. In this case, head to bed early and let the final hours of the fast be completed in your dreams. When you wake up the next day, it will be time to feast.

Your breakfast should be a few pieces of fruit. They are easy for you to digest and will also provide you with a good dose of energy. This is the best part of fasting. Food somehow tastes so much better after the 32 hours. You will appreciate eating so much more, and within a few hours, you will start to feel the energy pulsing through you. It enlightens you by showing you food is a potent source of fuel that enables you to control your body. During this first meal, don't overeat or you might irritate your stomach since you haven't digested any food for some time. After eating your fruit, wait 30 minutes, and then you can start eating regularly again. At this point, your fast is complete. It's not an easy task, but there are several benefits to fasting, making it well worth the effort.

Fasting Benefits

Abstaining from food has many benefits. Keep them in mind when you are going through your fast. It will help you persevere when water no longer seems to be enough.

1. Fasting allows you to lose a massive amount of body fat. The day you fast, you will consume 0 calories, and this will have a substantial effect. Your body requires between 1800 to 2500 calories a day just to maintain itself. While fasting, you don't add any calories to your system, so your body needs to use your reserve of energy to keep you alive and functioning. It starts by using up all the left-over energy from sugars and carbs. When that's depleted, it will start using your fat storage. This will begin around 12 to 16 hours into the fast. There is no precise time when it starts, as every person is different. Therefore, it's essential to continue the fast until you reach the 32-hour mark to benefit from this effect fully.

2. It's also a fantastic way to get rid of bloating. When you are bloated, you might be feeling pressure in your stomach.

It feels as if something is pushing it out. When you stop eating for 32 hours, the pressure will completely go away, and your stomach will feel genuinely empty. In time, if it returns, you can take this as a cue that it's time to start another fast. If you have ever experienced this discomfort before, now you know the solution.

3. It can remove the fog from your mind, and you will think more clearly. It will feel as if a curse has been lifted and your thoughts are free to roam as they please. This effect is most observable in the morning when you eat breakfast at the end the of the fast. The next day after you finish, you will be more focused and more motivated than you have ever been. It's honestly a beautiful feeling and one that you will experience for yourself.

4. It improves your metabolism and your digestion. It gives your stomach some rest for a day, and this allows it to reset itself. You will have better bowel movements and be able to burn fat more efficiently. Your body uses a lot of energy to metabolize your food every day. When you abstain from digestion, your body uses that excess energy to recover and heal. Your skin may clear up, and it's not uncommon for red spots to vanish overnight after a fast.

5. When you complete your first fast, you will come to realize how much your body depends on food for energy. It's one of the most significant revelations that fasting will bestow upon you. You realize how much power is packed in the food you eat. It's your fuel, and when you deprive yourself of it even for 32 hours, you quickly lose a lot of your human powers. Your legs will feel weak; your brain will not be as sharp as it is when you are eating. Embrace this feeling and learn from it; it has much to teach you.

6. It counts as a green square on your calendar. It's not a physical activity, but because it helps you lose weight, it counts. Fasting is terrific for your health and is an integral part of your weight loss journey. Write it on your calendar in green and use the blue marker as well. It counts as something extra since it requires the entire day.

Symptoms

You may experience some symptoms when you fast. You should recognize them when they appear, so you can be ready to deal with them. There is no need to be afraid; they are a regular part of the fasting process.

1. The first time you might get a mild headache or dizziness. Drink a tall glass of water and go lie down for a few

minutes. When you get up, do it slowly, or you might start seeing black dots. If this happens, just sit back down and drink a glass of water. Wait a minute and then get up slowly.

2. Not eating might cause you to be irritable. If you can, avoid any stressful activity during your fast. As I mentioned before, try to begin on one of your days off so you can better manage your emotions and avoid stress.

3. Be aware your reactions and thoughts might be slightly affected. You might be a bit slower than usual and not as sharp. You might experience fatigue and lack of focus when you stop eating for 32 hours. Remember to do the least amount of physical activity to avoid feeling overly fatigued. Also, don't plan any big projects or anything that requires your full attention, as it's not only fatigue of the body but of the mind as well. You can take a nap during the day; this will help restore some energy.

4. Fasting can cause bad breath. This happens because, without any daily meals, you will produce less saliva. Your saliva helps fight bacteria that cause bad breath. It's not something you should worry about, but you may want to consider it before kissing your significant other.

What Not to Do

You should wait until you have successfully passed the fasting step before even attempting to do it during work hours. I have fasted at my workplace but only after successfully doing it at home. I work in an office and sit the entire day, yet I still find it hard to do my job while fasting. Even though I know what to expect, it's hard to stay focused. I rarely fast at work anymore because I had a terrible experience one time. The start of the day was going smoothly, but then it got hectic in the afternoon, and I was having a tough time coping with the stress, focusing on the job and managing my hunger. I ended up stopping the fast and went to get a sandwich at the cafeteria. This is one of the only times I ever quit a fast. I didn't want to risk being angry with a client or losing my patience. If you do a physical job like construction, for example, I don't recommend you ever fast at work. You don't want to get light-headed and injure yourself or someone else.

When abstaining from food, don't do any extraneous physical activity like biking, running or any other sports. Moving your body in any way requires energy, and you will have very little to spare. Food provides you with your daily dose of energy, but since you are not eating, you need to avoid spending energy. The more active you are, the more the body will demand food and the hungrier you will get. It will then become much harder to continue the fast. If

46

you must, you can do light activity such as walking. You can also do simple tasks such as cleaning, doing the laundry or small household chores. Try to avoid doing anything that would typically make you exhausted or sweaty. Instead, read a book, watch some television or go sit outside, but don't do any heavy lifting. This is the only time you can do nothing, yet your fat will still melt off so take advantage of it.

You must never cheat because when you fast, your body stops digestion completely. If you eat anything, your digestion will start up again, and it defeats the entire purpose, and your previous sacrifice will have been done in vain. The longer you go without food, the more your body will use up your fat reserves. When you start the digestive system because you eat something, even something small, that automatic fat-burning process will stop and your fast will have failed. Make sure to pick an appropriate time to fast and avoid succumbing to food temptation.

You should avoid cooking any food. Being near food will make it that much hard to resist eating.When you must prepare food for others, be mindful of your every movement because you might be tempted to taste the food subconsciously. This desire will be even stronger now that you are fasting. I have spit food out on numerous occasions because I caught myself eating subconsciously.

Fun Facts

- Humans have been fasting for thousands of years, mostly as part of spiritual practices performed by Hindus, Christians, Jews, Buddhists, and Muslims. It has been part of the human tradition for a millennium.
- Animals instinctively fast when they are sick to give more power to the immune system to fight off the disease.
- Some people have been able to fast for over 700 hours, so don't worry about not eating for 32 hours.

At the beginning of humanity, people had to hunt and gather food. Somedays, they wouldn't eat for lack of food, but the next night, they would feast after a kill. Famine was an on-going threat to the survival of early man. This pattern of scarcity prompted the body to adapt and store excess food in the form of fat. This fat was then burned for energy during periods of starvation. Humans have survived for thousands of years because of this capacity to store substantial amounts of fat.

Your body inherited this natural mechanism, which you can now take full advantage of through fasting. When you abstain from eating, you will start to use up your fat reserve as the prime source of fuel to power your body. This is the most natural way to burn off this excess fat. The body stores fat for this very reason. All you must do is give it the right conditions, and it will burn the fat for you. This is what fasting is all about.

In today's world, you might never run out of food, and in fact, you have more than you need in so many different varieties. Your basic human instinct wants you to eat all the time. Your mind is still hard-wired to eat as much food as possible because of this "safety measure," which is meant to protect you in times of starvation. When famine never comes, you just accumulate more and more fat. You must use your mind and make an intelligent choice not to eat in excess knowing there will always be more food later.

The Challenges

1. Successfully complete a 32-hour water fast.
2. Don't cheat by eating food or drinking any calories.

I recommend you fast once a month. If you decide you're comfortable to fast twice a month, leave a 2-week period in-between to give yourself time to recover fully. Once you have finished step four, you will have successfully completed the hardest stage of your journey. Continue to fast, and you will be amazed by the results that will follow. You are now ready to move on to step 5.

STEP 5: THE BICYCLE

On this step, I will ask you to replace one of your weekly walks with a bike ride. Once a week, instead of walking, take your bike and go for a 1-hour trip. This will count as a green square on your calendar as any walk would. The goal of this step is to do something different than walking to shake things up and have some fun.

If you're already biking, this will be a natural step for you. If you have never ridden a bike before, use this as an opportunity to learn. You can learn a new sport, no matter what your age, weight or fears are. All you need is to channel your will to do it. Use your weight loss goal to motivate you to push forward. You have accomplished so much already.

I strongly recommend you try biking, but if for some reason you can't bike, any other sport will due. You can start playing tennis, hockey, basketball, soccer, roller-skating or any other sport. The point of this step is to start using your new body for something other than walking. I chose biking because it's a beautiful sport that I love, and almost anyone can do it. It's also an excellent introduction to sports in general and has numerous benefits, as you will see.

You are stronger now than ever before. Eliminating white sugar, walking almost every day and fasting has started to pay off. Having shed some body fat, you are now lighter on your feet. Because of your daily walks, your legs are getting stronger, making every movement easier. Your energy level will have improved by adding more fruits to your diet. Thus, bicycling should be easier for you now. Take on this new step with self-assurance. Adding cycling to your life will be like offering yourself a well-deserved gift. There are several reasons why cycling is a beautiful addition to your weekly routine.

- It's one of the best cardiovascular workouts you can do, and it provides an alternative from your regular walks.
- You can do it by yourself, eliminating the need to coordinate with others on a specific day to play a sport.
- You can do it all year long by using a stationary bike during winter months. You can cycle outside during winter months, but make sure to have the right tires.
- It's also a means of transportation. You can bike to work, school or to around town instead of taking your car. Thus, you will save money on gas and get your exercise done for the day. Instead of sitting in your car, you can now use this time to lose weight and get your green square. If you live in a city with a lot of traffic, biking can even be faster than driving.

Before you go out and start pedaling, I will give you a refresher on the fundamentals of cycling. I have put together the basics everyone should know. I will guide you to choose the right bicycle for you. I will teach you how to keep your bike in top shape. I will explain how to lock it properly to discourage potential thieves and how to find the best routes for your new ride. Let the biking adventure begin.

Choosing Your Bicycle

Unless you already have one, you must obtain a bicycle. There are several types of bikes, and each has their own purpose. I will go over the three most common bicycles you will find on the market. They are the mountain bike, the hybrid, and the road bike.

They come in all price ranges. There are two main factors that influence the price of the bike. The type of material used in the frame and the quality of the parts that make up the rest of the bike. Less expensive frames are made of steel, and the more expensive ones will be made of aluminum or carbon. They are all excellent frames, but aluminum and carbon are much lighter. The lightweight materials enable the bike to go faster, and they are easier to transport. Your budget and the type of terrain you intend to bike on should guide you to the correct choice.

Mountain bikes are designed for off-road riding. The price starts at around $100. The wheel is thicker than on a hybrid bike or a road bike. This gives you more grip on the road but will make it harder to pedal. All-terrain bicycles usually have suspension on the front, which adds weight to the bike but creates a smoother riding experience. If you intend to do some off-roading, this is the bike for you.

The hybrid is the middle ground between a mountain bike and a road bike. It costs between $250 to $1000 for a good hybrid bike. The fundamental differences are that the handlebars are straight. This is a more traditional position intended for comfort, not speed. The tires are thinner than the mountain bike. It is easier to pedal on roads than the previous bikes yet not as light or fast as the road bike. The hybrid bike is an excellent choice if you live in a city and want to commute to work. It's terrific entry bicycle to the sport, but it tends to be a bit more expensive than a standard mountain bike.

The road bike is the most expensive of the three. It starts at around $600 and can go up to $5000. It's the lightest bike, and it is designed for speed and performance. It's meant to achieve maximum performance on the road. The handlebars curve down, allowing for several hand placements. The seating position you take on the bike tends to be very horizontal to provide the least amount of wind resistance. There is no suspension or any other heavy components to slow you down. The tires are very narrow and have minimal tread, making it ideal for the road, but it provides little traction in off-road situations. This is a good option if you want to achieve top speed and have some cycling experience.

If you have a balance problem, you can always purchase an adult tricycle. They go for about $450 and can be a suitable alternative to a standard bike. You could also get a stationary bike. They are a terrific addition to your cycling life. You can use them during the winter or when it's raining outside.

If you don't have much money to spend, you might consider finding a used bicycle online. I have seen some for as low as $10 or even free. Often, these bikes will have problems that may need to be fixed. I don't recommend doing this unless you are able to do your own bike repairs.

Once you have chosen the type of bike you want, there are a few other things to keep in mind:
1. I recommend you acquire one that has 21 speeds. This allows you to adjust the tension, making it easier to pedal uphill and faster when going in a straight line.
2. You must find a bike with the correct frame length for your arms and body. A rule of thumb is. the taller you are, the

longer you want your frame to be.

3. Most importantly, try out the bike and see if you are comfortable riding on it. If your budget still allows, you might want to consider a few additional pieces of gear.

Optional Gear

Besides the bike, there are a few extra pieces of gear you can procure. The most important ones are a helmet, cycling gloves, a water bottle and pedal straps.

Wearing a helmet is the requirement by law in some cities. It protects your head in case of an accident. There are a few things to consider when buying a helmet: the airflow, the weight, and the size. It's essential to have good airflow in the helmet to ensure you don't overheat while wearing it. A lightweight helmet makes it more comfortable to wear for extended periods of time, causing less strain on your neck and making your ride more enjoyable. Light helmets are made of more expensive materials and cost more. Get the correct size because if it's loose and moves on your head, it doesn't provide you with any protection if you fall. Remember to protect your hands as well.

Comfortable cycling gloves are a fantastic addition to your gear. When you hold the handlebars for an hour or more, you can develop calluses on your palms. They can be painful, but the gloves will prevent this from happening. They also provide you with some added grip and protect your hands if you happen to fall off.

A water bottle is vital for every single ride you go on. As you exercise and sweat, you need to re-hydrate yourself to prevent getting dizzy or feeling sick. I recommend buying a decent quality water bottle that fits in a bracket you screw onto your bike frame. You can find these at your local bike shop.

Pedal straps are an excellent addition to your bicycle. They screw on to your pedals and go over your shoes, locking your feet into place while still permitting you to slide out if you need to stop. This allows you to pull the pedals as well as push down to advance, making it easier to pedal. It's also safer since there is no chance of you slipping off the pedal and hitting the frame, especially when biking upright.

All the gear above is optional but will help make your riding experience safer and more enjoyable. The items aren't expensive, so if your budget permits, get some extra gear for your new ride.

Bicycle Upkeep

Like a car, you must maintain your bike to keep it in working condition and ensure its lifespan. You need proper tire pressure, a well-oiled chain and a safe place to store it.

You must always check to make sure you have enough air in your tires before you go for a ride. The pressure required varies depending on the type of tire; it is measured in psi (pounds per square inch). Wider tires require less psi than narrow ones. Road tires need about 80 to 130 psi; mountain tires require between 25 to 40 and hybrid between 50 to 75. The necessary psi should also be noted on the side of the tire itself. You can use a gauge to measure the pressure or get an air pump that comes with one. If you don't have an indicator, a good trick is to press down on each of the tires with both of your thumbs. If you can push the tire in, add some air. The tire needs to be firm enough that you can barely push it in. The correct amount of air will give you a faster and smoother ride.

Always make sure your seat is at the correct height before leaving. Sit on your bike, and when your pedal is at the bottom and at the 6 o'clock position, your leg should be at a 30-degree angle. If it's not, put the seat up. If you can no longer touch the pedal, bring the seat down. It can be adjusted by loosening the screw around the seat pole and raising or lowering it.

Clean your bike chain and remove any debris that accumulates. Once cleared of debris, add some bicycle oil to it. A clean well-oiled chain is critical to the functionality of the bicycle. This should be done at least twice per season.

Store your bicycle inside if you can. If you must leave it outside, cover it with a tarp. Unlike a car, bicycle parts are fully exposed and will rust if left out in the rain. When your bike has rust, some moving parts will start to squeak. It also weakens the metal, making it more prone to breaking. If you leave it in the rain, make sure to wipe off all the water.

Bicycle Security

When leaving your bike for extended periods of time, you must always lock it securely. You will need to buy a decent quality lock to deter thieves. Then, you must find the best place to lock it up. You can do this by prioritizing the most expensive parts that are most likely to be stolen.

No lock is unbreakable, but high-quality ones will take more time to break into and require powerful, noisy tools to cut. Thieves want to avoid drawing attention to themselves and minimize the time they spend at the scene of a crime. They are looking for an easy score. If you present them with a challenging target, they will move on to the next one, and your bike will remain safe.

There are 3 types of bike locks: chain, U-lock, and cable locks. There are three key factors to consider when choosing a lock: the weight, the security it brings and the ease of locking and unlocking it.

Chain locks are the most secure of the 3, but they are also the heaviest. It is hard for thieves to cut through because of the thick chainlinks and the way the chain moves when attempting to saw it off. It's easy to use since you can twist it and pass it around the wheels and frame. The downside of this lock is the weight; it's around 10 pounds. A chain lock is a great option if you can handle the load. People tend to wear them across their chest to manage the bulk more efficiently. They go for around $30 to $100.

U-locks are a good middle ground option. They're not as heavy and provide excellent security, but they can be harder to lock up. I recommend the U-lock as it's an excellent middle range between safety and weight. Most U-locks and chain locks will require power tools and time to cut through. It comes in at around 3 pounds. You can find them for as cheap as $14, but high-quality ones go for about $40.

The cable lock is the weakest one but the lightest and most straightforward to use due to its length and flexibility. It's the least expensive, but they won't provide you with much security. It can quickly be snapped with a good pair of bolt cutters. It should be your last resort when locking a bike. Cable locks can still be used if you are locking your bike in a safe area like on your property or if you have it with you as an emergency lock. No matter what lock you choose, if you leave your bike in the wrong place, it might not be there when you come back.

A bicycle parking rack is the best place to attach your bike. Some are even monitored by cameras. If you can't find one, lock it on a busy public street to something secure. Don't try and hide your bike and lock it in a hidden place. Contrary to what you might think, it's better to have more people around. A thief will be less likely to saw off a lock in a public place. When you have found your spot, always prioritize locking the frame, then the back wheel and finally the front wheel, if you still have enough length on your lock. The frame is the most expensive part of the bike, and so it must be the priority. Once your bike is locked correctly, you will have peace of mind. Now that you know the basics, you're ready to find the path.

Bicycle Path

The best place to start is on a dedicated bicycle trail. Nature trails should be at the top of your list. You get to see beautiful plants and animals. I recommend you go online and look at Google Maps to find out all the bike trails in your city. Find one that appeals to you and head for it. If there are none in your area, you can just take your bike out for a spin around the neighborhood.

Bike paths are located everywhere: by the water, among trees and right on the streets. They are the most convenient way to travel. You should always prioritize roads that have them to avoid having to ride beside cars. You won't have to watch out for traffic or breathe in the nasty pollution expelled by gas-powered vehicles. If possible, steer clear of big boulevards and stick to the small streets. Even if it means a slight detour, it's worth it.

Motivation

If you're feeling demotivated to start, stand up and affirm out loud your exercising intentions. Command your body to do the task at hand. For example: "Get up now and start bicycling!" This may sound crazy, but it will help you to get motivated. Commanding yourself out loud makes the request more real for yourself and in your mind. This is another tool to help you fight procrastination and to get you up.

A timer can also enhance your motivation and focus your mind. Activate the timer and set it for 60 minutes. Your brain will create a link with the beginning of the timer and the start of your ride. You will feel an urge to start bicycling. Subconsciously, you don't want to be late, not even to your own workout. Before you know it, you will be done. There are 24 hours in a day, so one hour a day to maintain your body for the next 100 years is a tiny price to pay.

The Challenges

1. Obtain a bicycle.
2. Find a bike path.
3. Replace one of your walks each week with biking.

I love to bicycle on a bright sunny day. It feels wonderful to feel the wind on my face created by the power of my legs. I pedal as fast as I can and stand on my bike, letting it push me forward effortlessly. For a few seconds, I feel like a bird gliding in the sky, free of worry or concern, free of myself and of my surroundings. For a few seconds, I am riding the wind, and it sings in my ears, a deafening tune of peace and harmony.

Your biking perception may differ from mine. It can be a simple exercise tool you use to help you lose weight. It can be a means of transportation to go to work, a hobby you enjoy or a passion that can change your life. As you start bicycling, your view on it may change with time and improve. Give it a chance and let yourself enjoy this fabulous invention. Hopefully, you can enjoy it as much as I do and lose some weight doing it. Once you have biked 4 times a month, you can move on to the next step.

STEP 6: EATING BETTER

You must always be vigilant about any food you consume. What you eat has the power to transform your body into a fat-burning machine or a fat-absorbing blob. You have already gone through some food changes. In step one, you changed from white sugar to fruits. Now on the sixth step, your focus will be on eating better in a more general sense. First, I will share with you some tips and tricks regarding how to eat and to avoid overeating. Second, you will learn to eat foods that will make you feel full and help you lose weight. This will include swapping bad carbs for good ones, adding more vegetables to your meals and alternating your protein consumption. Food has an enormous impact on your weight, so it's essential you understand it's role in your everyday life.

Calorie Awareness

It's important to understand that a calorie is a unit of energy. One calorie is the amount of energy required to raise one gram of water by one degree Celsius. Our body uses calories in the same way a car uses fuel to move. When you digest food, your body transforms it into energy that is used to power your heart, your legs and every other part of your body. You need between 1600 to 3000 calories daily depending on your sex, height, age and many other factors. How many calories each person needs is highly debated. Plus, the way food calories are calculated lacks precision and is usually more of an approximation. Thus, it's almost impossible to attain the correct numbers for either. Therefore, I don't recommend you track every single calorie since the information lacks the accuracy it would need to be useful.

Instead, I want you to have a general idea of how many calories are in certain foods. You can do this by reading food labels and going online to verify the calorie content of the foods you eat the most. Eventually, you'll know the energy content of most of your meals. You might be surprised to notice that some foods bring you no health benefits but add a lot of calories to your snacks and meals. At this point, you can then make an informed decision to keep certain foods while discarding others. You might end up eating more in the end but ingesting fewer calories. This is the goal.

Be careful when reading food nutrient labels; they can be misleading. Sometimes, what is listed is only a portion of what the container holds. For example, a can of soup may contain 750 ml, but the label is showing you the nutrient value for 250 ml, so you need to multiply it by 3 to get the correct number of calories for the entire can. It can get tricky at times, so keep an eye on it.

Controlled Consumption

Overeating is a significant factor that influences your weight, and it's a difficult habit to break. There are several reasons why you do this and understanding them is how you will be able to overcome this obstacle. In this section, you will learn 4 tricks that will assist you in this task: Only look at food if you are hungry, eat slowly, eat from smaller plates and don't be afraid to leave food on your plate.

Stop seeking food if you're not hungry. When you see food, your brain already sends a message to your stomach to start preparing itself for digestion. In other words, the sight of food provokes hunger. Only look for food if you are hungry, or you might find yourself in front of the refrigerator eating when your belly is already full. Before you go looking for food, ask yourself the following questions:

- When was the last time I ate? If you just ate a few minutes ago, give yourself some time for your brain to receive the message that you are full. If you are still hungry in 30 minutes, have a snack high in fiber, like a banana, to satiate you.
- When was the last time you had a drink of water? If you haven't had a glass of water in the previous hour, it's possible your only thirsty. Have a glass of water and wait 15 minutes and see if your hunger doesn't dissipate.

Slowly Eating will help you consume less food and provide time for your brain to get the "I'm full" message. Otherwise, you might overeat and consume all those unnecessary calories. Stomach pains can follow, but they can be prevented if you slow down. So, aim to eat as slowly as possible. I have a few tips to help you with this:

- Chew your food 5 to 10 times before swallowing. This will slow down your eating pace, plus it makes the food easier to digest for your stomach.

- Another good tip is to avoid eating alone. Eat with others when possible and engage them in conversation. This will help focus your mind on something besides the food. If you are eating faster than them, stop eating until they have as much food left as you do. Match their slower speed of eating and see if you can let them finish eating before you.

- For each bite, load less food on your fork. Pick your food slowly and make each bite count. Wait until you have swallowed before picking up more with your fork. This will improve the entire eating experience, and you should eat less in the process.

- Some people tend to devour their food if they are enjoying the meal. Be mindful of this when eating your favorite dish. Since you love it, take your time and savor it.

The size of your plates and bowls directly impacts the amount of food you tend to serve yourself for one portion. Use smaller dishes; subconsciously, you will put less food on your plate and thus eat a reduced amount. This is due to a tendency to fill empty space. If you use larger dining wear, you will tend to serve yourself more food to fill up the empty plate, thus eating more. As a dining rule, smaller is always better.

Leave food on your plate. You must break the habit of finishing food because it's in front of you. If you are unsure, ask yourself the following question: am I eating because I'm still hungry or because it's delicious? This will confirm if you are eating out of hunger or gluttony. If it's hunger, wait 15 minutes and see if you are still hungry. If it's out of gluttony, save yourself the extra pounds and put the leftovers in the fridge. Not only will you eat fewer calories, but you will get to enjoy the meal again tomorrow.

You may have this misconception that it's impolite to leave food on your plate or that someone's feelings will get hurt if you refuse food. This could not be further from the truth. In fact, some cultures see uneaten food as a sign that you ate to your satisfaction. So, if someone offers you more food but you're not hungry, just say, "No thank you. It was delicious."

You must control and take responsibility for all the food you eat. Don't let anyone else make that decision for you. It's easy to blame others instead of taking responsibility for your overeating. Make a vow now to be responsible for everything that goes into your mouth. Controlling how much you eat is only half the battle;

now, you must adjust what you eat.

Introduction to Carbohydrates

Bread has a special place in my heart. It's my favorite food, and I have been eating it happily my entire life. During my weight loss journey, I cut it out entirely after I learned how much weight I could lose from abstaining from bread, pizza, rice, and pasta. I was surprised at how quickly I started to lose weight. I love bread, so I eventually incorporated it back into my diet, but I made a necessary change. I now only consume whole wheat sugar-free bread as opposed to refined white bread. This is a portion of what I want you to do.

As part of step six, you need to replace bad carbohydrates with good ones. There has been a lot of controversy over the last few years about carbs. Will they make you gain weight or lose weight? The answer is, they can do both. If you eat good carbs or whole carbohydrates, you will most likely lose weight. If you eat bad carbs or refined carbs, you will most likely gain weight. You need to identify the bad carbs you are consuming daily, so you can replace them with good ones. You already eliminated sugar products in step one so that won't be covered here. Before you can start, you need to understand what carbs are and how to identify each one.

Identifying Carbs

So, what are carbs? Carbohydrates are a category of food. They consist of the fibers, sugars, and starches found in many foods. They consist of approximately 50% of what most people eat. They come in many shapes and forms, and new ones are created every year. They can be both good and bad for you. Since they come from a vast family of food, it can be hard to make the distinction between the good carbs and the bad ones. I will explain some of the critical differences and show you some examples to guide you towards the light. Once you have learned the truth, you will need to replace the bad carbs with good ones.

Whole carbohydrates are the good ones. They are the fruits, vegetables, beans, brown rice, quinoa and many more. Anything that is unmodified and looks like it just came from the earth is a good carb. You might wonder why they are better than refined carbs. There are a few reasons for this:
- They are low in saturated fats.
- They have no added sugar or refined grains.
- They are high in fiber and nutrients.
- You will feel full while consuming fewer calories.

Refined carbs are the bad ones. They are found in white bread, white rice, white pasta, pastries, fruit drinks, chips, candy and more. They have been refined to have all nutrients and fibers removed. This process creates products that have virtually no health benefits, only empty calories. These products are the leading cause of obesity and diabetes. The goal of such food is not to feed you but to keep you hungry asking for more. Most refined carbs are:

- High in saturated fats.
- Have added sugar.
- Low in fiber and nutrients.
- Empty calories with no nutritional benefits.

Replace Bad with Good

Bad Carbs	Good Carbs
White bread, bagels, croissants	Whole wheat, rye, spelt bread and oatmeal
White rice	Brown rice or quinoa
Pasta, pizza	Vegetables
Potato chips	Popcorn, nuts: almonds, walnuts, peanuts, and pumpkin seeds
Mayonnaise and BBQ sauce	Hot sauce and mustard

Bad Carbs

1. **White bread** is the staple of bad carbs. The wheat used in white bread is completely transformed in the manufacturing process, causing most of the nutrients to be discarded. This

71

has a two-part effect. First, it will force you to eat more since it has fewer fibers to make you satiated. Second, white bread has added sugar, so you crave it more to fill your sugar need as you saw in Step 1.

2. **Chips** are one of the most popular snacks and part of almost everyone's daily eating habits. It's important to minimize the impact snacks can have on your weight loss quest. It's easy to fall into a bag of chips and finish it, not realizing you just ate about 1000 to 2000 calories. Chips are one of the worst refined carbs on the market and should be avoided at all cost.

3. **Mayonnaise** is one of the highest calorie condiments on the market at 50 calories per tablespoon. This is a considerable amount when you realize most sandwiches contain at least 3 tablespoons. So when eating a lunch made with mayo, you are eating more calories from the condiments than from the bread. Think about that next time, before you spread it on both slices. You might want to trade that white fat for some wholesome, yellow mustard.

Good Carbs

1. **Mustard** has a unique taste and has virtually no calories, standing proudly at 3 calories per tablespoon. It even helps prevent cancer and control diabetes on top of keeping you

slimmer. Try different varieties of mustard and find one that suits your taste.

2. **Brown rice** is an excellent alternative to white rice. It's much healthier for you and will help you lose weight. It has loads of fiber, which will make you satiated. Thus, you will be less likely to eat more after your meal.

3. **Popcorn** is a great crunchy snack. It's very healthy and has only 30 calories per cup. Avoid buying bags of premade popcorn as they contain added calories. Instead, use an air blown machine to make your own, as they don't require any oil. Sprinkle some salt on it for a great low-calorie snack.

4. **Nuts and seeds** are an excellent snack choice. Most have their share of fat, but they have many other benefits, including protein. They also satiate you, causing you to eat less. Give them a try and see which one you prefer. You can choose from peanuts, almonds, walnuts, sunflower seeds, and pumpkin seeds, just to name a few.

5. **Hot sauce** is delicious and has almost no calories. It stands at 3 to 5 calories per tablespoon compared to 25 to 30 calories for barbecue sauce. The capsaicin found in hot sauce raises your metabolism which will cause you to burn more fat. It also increases your level of satiety by making you eat less. If you're not used to spicy food, then it will take some getting used to. Start with small amounts at first

and mix it with mustard to alleviate the spiciness.

6. **Oatmeal** is a fantastic addition to any breakfast and can replace your refined carbs. It's made of whole grains and will give you energy throughout the day as it's slowly digested. It also coats the interior of your stomach and protects it for the rest of the day. It's low in fat and high in fiber, so you'll still stay satiated longer and consequently, you will eat less during the day.

7. **Whole wheat bread** is a better choice than any white variety. It has more fiber and has no added sugar. There is also rye bread, spelt bread, and wheat-free brands. Give it a try, and over time, you might prefer them for their nutty taste. Aim to eat no more than 2 slices a day.

These are only a few of the most common examples among the thousands of carbs out there. To summarize, good carbs have fiber, are natural and make you feel full. Bad carbs are transformed, have very little fiber and leave you hungry, wanting more. Always be mindful of what you eat and start replacing some of your bad carbs with good ones. It's up to you to eliminate bad carbs and let the good ones bring you closer to your weight loss goal. Choose your foods wisely, and your body will see that you are rewarded. When eating vegetables or other good carbs, you can devour your food without guilt or regret.

Vegetables

As part of step six, you need to incorporate more vegetables into every meal. When trying to lose weight, plants are the most important food to eat. This is because most of them contain an insignificant number of calories. Therefore, it's almost impossible to gain weight when eating veggies, so you can eat them without restraint. They also supply all the vitamins, minerals and fibers the body needs. Fibers help you feel full and are an excellent tool for weight loss. Some vegetables are healthier than others, but it's better you choose the ones you enjoy since you are more likely to stick with them. Remember, you are eating to fill your body's need for nourishment but also to enjoy the experience. Always strive to find a way to do both and avoid leaving one out.

You will need to make a list of vegetables and buy them every week. Add the ones you already enjoy to the list. It should contain at least 5 vegetables to start with. Tastes vary between individuals so you will need to experiment and choose the ones that suit you best. Before long, you will have an extensive list of produce. Your checklist will contain all the vegetables you should have handy in your kitchen. Now that you have your list, it's important to know how to choose quality products.

Knowing how to pick vegetables at the supermarket will ensure you get tasty veggies. Unripe vegetables will usually taste bitter or sour. Rotten vegetables will have a repulsive taste and can even make you sick. As a general guideline, you want to avoid anything that has a bruise on it, brown spots, white moss, dark discoloration or that offers little resistance when pressed. These are warning signs that a vegetable is about to expire. Instead, choose the ones that have the brightest color, uniformity, and firmness. By following this simple rule, you will buy quality products to create an excellent meal.

There are so many delicious vegetables to choose from. Each has their own health benefits and qualities. I encourage you to try a new vegetable every week to discover your favorite one. I have put together a small list to get you started.

1. **Bell peppers** are sweet and add some crunchiness for a savory meal. At 45 calories per cup, you can eat as much as you want without feeling guilty. Specific enzymes and vitamins in the sweet pepper protect your eyes and skin against disease.

2. **Broccoli** is high in fiber and low in fat. At around 30 calories per cup, it can fill you up with no added weight gain. It will also lower your cholesterol and fight cancer on your behalf.

3. **Carrots** are the food of visionaries; the beta-carotene helps maintain your eyesight. They only have about 50 calories

per cup. When refrigerated, they can last for several weeks. When eating them raw, stay away from high-calorie dips. Instead, accompany them with a healthy alternative such as guacamole, olive oil or hummus, which are delicious and healthy for you.

4. **Celery** has one of the lowest calorie counts at 16 calories per cup. It's packed with fiber that helps you become satiated. It's filled with antioxidants, anti-inflammatory properties, and vitamin K.

5. **Lettuce** has nearly no calories, and it's almost impossible to run out of recipes to use it in. You can mix in bell peppers for a delicious side dish or add some proteins like chicken or beans to make a complete meal. You should avoid adding high-calorie dressing. Instead, mix some olive oil and balsamic vinegar to make a low-fat dressing.

6. **Avocado** is a vegetable filled with fat and has about 350 calories. Believe it or not, it's great for helping you lose weight. On top of lowering your cholesterol, it decreases your appetite, making you eat less after consuming it. A fantastic way to eat it is as a dip. Just slice it in half, remove the pit and scoop out the rest. Crush it with a fork and mix it with salsa or spicy sauce. You then have a delicious dip for your vegetables, or you can spread it on toast.

7. **Onions** are a great addition to any meal. You can mix them

in brown rice or cook them alongside other vegetables. They have 45 calories per cup. They are well-known for their healing benefits and help prevent certain types of cancer. As you get older, your taste buds change, so it's essential to give your blacklist foods a second chance. As a child, I hated onions, so I would avoid them like they were poison. I refused to eat whatever dish they were in. As I started eating healthier, I decided to try them again. I realized that onions didn't taste as nasty as I had remembered. In fact, they are sweet, crunchy and delicious. Open your mind to the possibility of enjoying a vegetable that you once hated.

Vegetables have always seemed like a magical food to me—small seeds that grow into a beautiful plant and produce all manner of colorful food. Through fire and heat, they can be transformed into a delicious meal that has properties to heal and maintain your body. They are a miracle of nature and will always be at your disposal to assist you in your weight loss journey.

Protein

As part of step six, I will ask you to alternate eating natural proteins and animal proteins. This will help cut down on the high amount of fat that comes with eating a lot of meat. Proteins are found in vegetables, nuts, dairy products and animal meat. When trying to lose weight, eating proteins will help you feel satiated because they take time to digest. Proteins make up the entire human body and are essential to your survival. They are used to repair the cells of the body and to make new ones. So, it's important not to neglect them. Here is a list of healthy proteins to get you started.

On the days you eat animal protein, select the ones that have less fat such as chicken, turkey, and fish. Avoid anything that comes from beef or pork, like steak, bacon, and ham, as they are high in fats.

- **Tuna** is an excellent choice on the animal side. It's low in fat but still packed full of protein. One cup of tuna holds about 180 calories and contains 95% protein and only 5% fat. When you eat canned tuna, make sure to remove all the water before consuming, or it will taste foul.
- **Turkey** has very little fat for animal meat when eaten without the skin. About 60% of turkey is protein, and 10% of it is fat. It's not as good as tuna, but it is an excellent alternative to a steak that has 30% fat. Turkey is healthy as it helps to lower your cholesterol.
- **Chicken** is one of the most eaten and popular meats in the world. If eaten without the skin, chicken has about 4 times more protein than fa keeping you satiated. Thus you will avoid overeating.

- **Eggs** are an excellent way to start your day, and they give you all the energy you need to power through the afternoon. They are loaded with protein, so they will keep you full for several hours.

When you eat natural protein, there are several to choose from. You can find protein in nuts yogurt and all kinds of different vegetables. Here a few of my personal favorites that I have stuck with throughout my weight loss journey.

- **Almonds** have shown to help you lose belly fat, and they are a great snack on the go. Although they can be expensive, they are worth the price. You don't need to eat many of them to feel full so avoid eating more than 10 in one sitting as they do hold their share of fat. Each almond has 7 calories, and 70% of that is fat.

- **Kale and spinach** are also packed with protein. They will help your muscles heal and grow. Kale is one of best foods on earth because it's packed with essential nutrients the body needs.

- **Greek yogurt** is a fantastic source of protein. It can be eaten as a dessert or a delicious snack. It has double the amount of protein of regular yogurt. It has 10 grams of protein for every 100 grams of yogurt and contains almost no fat. Avoid the ones that have added sugar.

Proteins will always remain an essential part of any diet. They keep you satiated and your body
fully repaired and functional.

The challenges

1. Avoid overeating.
2. Replace bad carbs with good ones.
3. Incorporate vegetables into most meals.
4. Alternate your protein consumption.

Give yourself one to two months to fully adapt to all these recent changes. These new habits will become easier the more you practice them, so do so every day. Focus on one change at a time and when you have accepted it in your daily life, see if you can add another one. Once you have added all of them, you will be ready to move on to the last step of your weight loss journey.

STEP 7: START RUNNING

On this last step, I will ask you to introduce some light running to your walks. I will explain a straightforward method I use that is simple and provides excellent results. I will go over all the benefits running will bestow upon you, some precautions you can take to avoid the most common injuries, and the importance of fluids. Don't worry if you haven't run for some time because it will be much easier now that you are lighter on your feet. It's time to get started.

How to Start

You must now add running to every single one of your walks. You will be engaging in what is referred to as run/walking. What this means is you will alternate between running and walking. When you go for your daily walk, start by walking for 2 to 5 minutes. Once you have warmed up, look for something further down the road, a stop sign, a cement block, a tree or a parked car. It can be any fixed object along your path. Fix that goal in your mind like it's the finish line to a race and run towards it. Once you reach it, touch the object and start walking again. It's important to place your hand on it to create a physical link with the achievement in your mind. When you are no longer exhausted, spot another object in the distance and repeat the process. Do this at least 3 times during your walk to complete your running cycle.

I recommend you start by jogging, then try running and finally go for a sprint at the end. There are some minor differences between the three styles of running, but the most significant variable is the pace.

- Jogging is done at a pace less than 10 km per hour. It's slightly faster than walking. Any quicker than that and you would be running. It's considered a low-intensity aerobic activity. Joggers will usually keep the same pace the entire time and will be able to maintain it for a more extended period. Due to the lower speed, jogging is safer, so you have less risk of injury. This style of running is an excellent place to start, but since you're only doing it for a brief period between walking, the weight loss rewards will be minor.

- Running is anything above 10 km per hour. It burns more calories than jogging, yet they are very similar. The main differences are the speed and the strides. When you run, you will be taking longer strides and pushing yourself more, thus rewarding yourself with greater fat burning. Running is more exhausting than jogging. Therefore, you may not be able to sustain it for prolonged periods of time. Running is the golden zone where you should aim to be.

- Sprinting is running as fast as you can over a brief period.

It's great for your body as it heightens your metabolism, promotes lean muscles and attacks the fat cells directly. It can easily be incorporated into the end of your run. At the end of your run, go for a quick sprint to spend your remaining energy and get some endorphins flowing in you.

Each time you go for a walk, see if you can run to the same object again or the equivalent distance. At first, you might be out of breath quickly, and your legs will tire easily; this is normal. Keep at it, even if you can only run for a few seconds. Eventually, it will become easier to run that distance as your lung capacity improves and you become less winded with each run. At this point, you can challenge yourself further and see if you can run past your goal and keep going. Look for a new location past the first one and run to it. Keep pushing yourself on every run and see how much more you can do. Remember, if you run more and run further, you will lose more weight.

The Benefits

You burn three times as many calories when you are running than when you are walking. This makes running one of the most effective ways to burn calories and lose weight. Alongside its significant weight loss benefits, running can also help if you have initial stages of diabetes or if you have high blood pressure. It lowers the risk of having a heart attack because running makes your heart stronger. It raises your good cholesterol and improves your immune system. It will enhance your overall lung function. The more you run, the more you will strengthen your entire body.

Your mind can also be healed by running. By completing your run/walk every day and getting to each finish line, you will be proud of yourself. You are proving to yourself daily that your body matters and you are doing actions towards your goal to achieve fitness. This daily success will improve your confidence and your self-esteem. Running can also help reduce your stress.

Doing cardio exercise is a natural stress reliever. If you are feeling stressed or depressed, running can easily remedy both those ailments. After running, when you are exhausted, your daily life pressures will shrink away into nothingness, and any negative feelings you might have will melt away like ice on a warm summer day. Your frown will be replaced by a broad smile on your face, and you will find peace of mind.

This is the result of your body releasing chemicals called endorphins, otherwise known as the "runner's high." This usually comes at the end of a run when having pushed yourself to the limit and exhausted all your energy. You will be out of breath, and your heart will be pounding. This is when you will feel that flow of endorphins that evaporates all negative emotions and replaces them with happiness and self-satisfaction. It's as if your body rewards you for having pushed yourself to the limit. It's your prize at the end of all your effort. You will feel like you're floating on a cloud. It's one of the best feelings the body can provide. Sometimes, it's the only reason you will go out there. All these benefits will be yours when you start putting on your running shoes and going for your daily dash.

Preventing Problems

They are some minor risks associated with running. I will go over the most common issues that can occur and how to prevent them. Most are due to bad form and improper footwear. Follow the indications below to avoid most injuries or discomforts.

Practicing correct form is essential for preventing aches and pains. Running can be hard on your body, especially on your knees and back. There are a few things you can do to avoid potential injury. You must maintain a proper form while jogging. Keep your upper torso straight and keep your head directly over your shoulders. This prevents adding stress to your knees and your back. Secondly, you should swing your arms slightly while you run. Bend them 90 degrees and keep your elbows close to your body. This will give you added stability.

Shoes are your most important piece of equipment. You should always run with the right pair on. You can run in boots or dress shoes, as I have done too often, but wearing the wrong shoe should always be avoided when possible. Over time, this can cause blisters, knee injuries, and back pain. This is a lesson I had to learn the hard way. Invest in a good pair of running shoes and plan to spend around $100.

When choosing a pair, always try several pairs to have something to compare to. Make sure your heel is snug but not tight. Your feet should never move within the shoe because if it does, you will develop blisters. The sneaker must be comfortable and literally feel like a part of your foot. You should never feel any tightness or pressure below the laces. In the front of your toes, you should always have a thumb's length in front of your longest toe. This will prevent most toe injuries. When you have found a pair that seems to be right, make sure to try them out and run around in them if possible. This will ensure you have bought the correct pair, and it will go a long way in preventing future problems. If you can follow these instructions, you will be on your way to obtaining a great pair of shoes, so you can start running on the right foot.

Hydration

Hydration is essential when you are running. The first sign of dehydration may present itself as a slight headache. When it gets worse, you may start to get muscle cramps and feel fatigued. It can also cause heart problems that can be dangerous. To prevent these symptoms, you must ensure you stay hydrated, even before you go out for a run. You don't need to calculate how much you drink. By listening to your body and drinking when thirsty, you should always be adequately hydrated. When you go out for a walk/run, bring some water with you and drink a few sips when you are thirsty. When you run, you sweat, so you lose more water than you would normally. Thus, you must drink more to replenish what is lost.

Every day you drink different beverages, but are you aware that some of them can help you lose weight? Many have almost no calories, but they are packed with some essential weight loss benefits, like speeding up your metabolism. I have listed the top beverages you should be drinking on a daily basis and some you should avoid that can hinder your weight loss mission.

Water is essential to life and to your weight loss journey. Always drink a glass of water when you get up in the morning. This will hydrate you and reduce the amount of food you will consume for breakfast. Water has 0 calories and will remain the best way to hydrate yourself. Always drink when you feel thirsty. This simple act will keep you hydrated and maintain your metabolism.

Sports drinks are beneficial to running. They replace the sodium and other minerals in your body that are sweated out of you during your exercise. They also provide a boost of energy in the form of carbohydrates. But, if you plan to run/walk for an hour, you will barely gain anything from them as you have not lost enough resources to value their consumption. Stick to water and only take a sports drink if you plan a long journey.

Lemon water adds some taste to your drink of water. On top of being delicious, it can:

- Improve digestion.
- Make skin beautiful.
- Boost your immune system.
- Fight cancer.
- Freshen breath.

Press a lemon to get all the juice out or buy a bottle of lemon juice. You can also add it to your tea instead of sugar.

Green tea has significant weight loss properties. Right before your run, drink some green tea. It boosts your metabolism, which helps burn more fat as you exercise, and it helps your body get rid of fat cells. It also has other health benefits including being high in anti-oxidants. Drink at least one cup of green tea a day.

Coffee speeds up your metabolism, which helps you lose weight. A cup of coffee is a great way to start your weight loss day. Just make sure you don't add any sugar to it. If you are having trouble drinking coffee with no sugar, try eating something sweet while you drink it, like a piece of your favorite fruit or add some 10% cream to your coffee. This will help to counteract the bitterness of the coffee while adding a silky texture.

Alcohol is one of the worst beverages you can choose before going for a run. It has a lot more calories than you might think, which is not always clear since most brands don't display the calorie content on the bottles. The exact amount of calories varies between brands. The type and the percentage of alcohol also plays a role in calories, but here is the general gist of it:

- A beer is about 150 calories.
- A glass of wine is around 120 calories.
- A shot of hard liquor has about 100 calories.

Thus, with regards to calories, having three or four drinks is equivalent to having a fourth meal. You can have a drink every few days but avoid having alcohol every day. When you do drink, limit yourself to one or two drinks to avoid adding all those unnecessary calories. But it's not just about the calories. Alcohol has a direct impact on how your body gets rid of fat.

It interferes with the body's fat-burning mechanism. This effect is known as fat sparing. When there is no alcohol in your system, your liver will metabolize your fat and turn it into energy for you to use, thus burning fat in the process. When you drink, your liver will use alcohol first to provide you with energy sparing your fat from being turned into energy thus leaving it to be stored on your body. This prevents you from losing weight and instead makes you gain additional pounds. Therefore, never drink alcohol before you exercise because this will prevent you from losing the fat you are sweating for.

Motivation

Sweating is a natural behavior of the human body you should never be ashamed of. On the contrary, be proud to be covered in sweat because it's a sign you did a full-body workout. Running will make you sweat very quickly as you use a lot of energy. The more you sweat, the more weight you will lose. So, every time you are soaking wet, imagine that it's the fat melting off you because, in a way, it is.

It can be intimidating to go out there and run for the first time in public. When you are outside running, don't worry about what people will think of you. Stay positive and focus on yourself and your movement to achieve a suitable form. People outside are going about their daily lives, and they're not concerned about what you are doing or why. Be proud of yourself and hold your head up high as you run past them.

As you start to lose weight, you might be tempted to think back on the past and regret not having started before. You might think to yourself; if you had started a year ago, you would be much slimmer today. This way of thinking is dangerous and will only lead to demotivation. You cannot change the past, but you can mold the future as you see fit. Do not dwell on what you cannot change. Instead, focus on what you can do in the present to better your future. A year from now, will you look back on today and tell yourself you should have started running or will you be proud that you did? Focus on the future and how much you will improve during the year. The past is over, but your future is always just beginning.

The Challenges

1. You must run at least 3 times during each of your daily walks for a month.
2. Try jogging, running and sprinting and find what is best for you.
3. Buy a good pair of running shoes.
4. Stay hydrated and try some alternatives to water.

When running becomes part of your daily routine, it will set you free from the confines of a prison made of fat. Your body is made to walk and run; it's not designed to sit down for prolonged periods. So, get moving and keep a positive image of yourself in mind. Running will not only cause you to lose weight, but it will also improve your state of mind and dissolve negative feelings. You will become slimmer, more relaxed, and free of stress. You will grow into your true self. Once you have run/walked for a month, you will have completed the last step of this book.

CONCLUSION

Congratulations on completing all the steps in *From Fat to Fit*. You have gone through some challenging obstacles to make it here, the finish line. This is a marvelous accomplishment and one that you should celebrate. Be proud of your achievement; even if your body is not perfect, it is healthier than it was when you started. The important thing is that you improved yourself. I invite you now to look at your body and see how much it has changed over the last few months. Look at one of the first pictures from your walks and see how much you have changed since you first started your journey.

It's vital that you continue using what you have learned during the steps to maintain your weight. You must hold true to them, so your body can keep up with your future adventures. You have lost some weight but remember, it's much easier to gain weight than it is to lose. Always keep your eye on the ball and continue to use the system. If you don't, the ball you will be looking at will be your bulging stomach returning.

Don't panic if you have a moment of weakness and go back to your old ways. This is likely to happen at some point, and it's to be expected. When this happens, you must pick up the tools I have given you in this book and put them in action. Here is a review of each step consisting of the principal elements to help you get back on track.

The Review

Step one: Continue to eat fruits and avoid consuming any source of white sugar. Avoid establishments that serve you sugar as a primary product. Don't keep any white sugar products in your home or office to prevent the temptation. Sugar is your worst enemy, and you must do all you can to avoid it. When you get a sugar craving, eat some fruit to help it pass. Remember, your body is only yearning sugar, and once you eat some in fruit form, the desire will quickly vanish. Always have a variety of fruits on hand to deal with the cravings.

Step two: Carry on with your daily walks and always go for one hour or more. This should now be part of your daily routine. Continue to take pictures while strolling; it will help you remember the positive side of your hour. Go out during your favorite time of day and always have a goal in mind before you step out the door. Check the weather right before each walk and gear up accordingly. Remember, you must never stop moving because your body is maintained by it. It doesn't matter if you're 20 years old or 60. People tend to blame time to justify their predicament, but time doesn't define your actions; only you can do that.

Step three: Continue to write on your calendar every day. This will keep you motivated and informed of your continual progress. Print out a new calendar every month and decorate it. Always be honest with it as it's a tool to reflect your growth. Good or bad, it will shine the light on what needs to be seen. Keep reading your green squares every week to motivate you. Read the red ones at the end of the month and see if a pattern emerges so you can find a solution. The calendar is a mighty tool, and you must continue to take advantage of its powerful visual representation of your progression.

Step four: Continue to fast every month. It will help maintain your body weight and keep your mind clear, so you can focus on your goal. Remember, during your fast, you cannot eat or drink any calories. Drink a lot of water during this time; it will make it much more comfortable. Only fast on your days off. Fasting is at the core of the system, and it's vital that you continue to do it.

Step five: Continue to bicycle once a week as a fun and useful alternative to walking. It will help you break the monotony and provide you with a simple alternative to cardio exercise. It serves as a mode of transport and saves you money on gas while getting your cardio done for the day. Remember to find a bicycle that suits your needs and keep it safe to avoid any negative experiences that might taint your view of cycling.

Step six: Eating right is essential to maintaining your body weight and health. Avoid overeating by not seeking food when you're not hungry and eating more slowly. Keep eating whole carbs while avoiding refined carbohydrates and continue to add vegetables to every meal. Continue to eat lean proteins to prevent excessive amounts of unwanted fat. You haven't failed if you eat a white burger bun, but don't let this become the norm or your will stray from the path.

Step seven: Running is the best way to lose those last persisting areas of fat. Do not underestimate its power in helping you achieve your goal. Keep running, the results may surprise you. Remember, running can also help you overcome depression, and it is a reliable tool for stress relief. Run with the proper shoes and the correct form and your weight loss will be a sure thing.

Last Words

You have gone through a lot these past few months. You have learned new techniques and tricks to get fit and lose weight. You must maintain your discipline and continue to walk on the path to healthiness.

One day, you will leave this earth, so don't rob yourself of the joy of living life to its full extent. No one is eternal, and so you must make the best of the little time you have on this big blue rock. Don't waste your time being out of shape and in pain, never being able to do the things you have always dreamed of doing with your life. I have given you all the tools you need to change your body. It's up to you to continue to use them and improve your quality of life.

Friends and family can be a source of motivation while you continue walking the steps. Once they have seen the positive results and how much weight you have lost, they will encourage you to keep it up. Tell the people closest to you about this adventure you embarked on so they can understand it and help you stay motivated in your continued efforts.

Keep doing what you're doing and let the steps be a new way of life for you. Embrace the changes that have come over your body and look forward to your future improvement. You now have all the tools necessary to maintain your body.

My work here is done. I have walked the steps with you and guided you as best as I can. It's up to you now to continue to use what you have learned. May your healthy body be with you, always.

100

Made in the USA
Las Vegas, NV
12 June 2023

73314581R00062